Dirty Little
Secrets

Dirty Little Secrets

Secrets

The Truth Behind The Door Called "Choice"

Vera Faith Lord

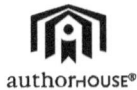

authorHOUSE®

AuthorHouse™
1663 Liberty Drive
Bloomington, IN 47403
www.authorhouse.com
Phone: 1-800-839-8640

First published by AuthorHouse   4/12/2010

ISBN: 978-1-4520-0659-8 (e)
ISBN: 978-1-4520-0660-4 (sc)

Printed in the United States of America
Bloomington, Indiana

This book is printed on acid-free paper.

THIS BOOK WOULD NEVER

HAVE BEEN WRITTEN WITHOUT

THE LOVE, HELP, & SUPPORT OF ---

Steven, Kevin, Olivia, Ernie,

Vicki, Barry, Diana, Michael

& first, last, & always,

Tim

THIS BOOK IS GOING TO MAKE YOU UPSET, shocked maybe even outraged. Good. It's about time. You've been lied to --- for decades. Wake up.

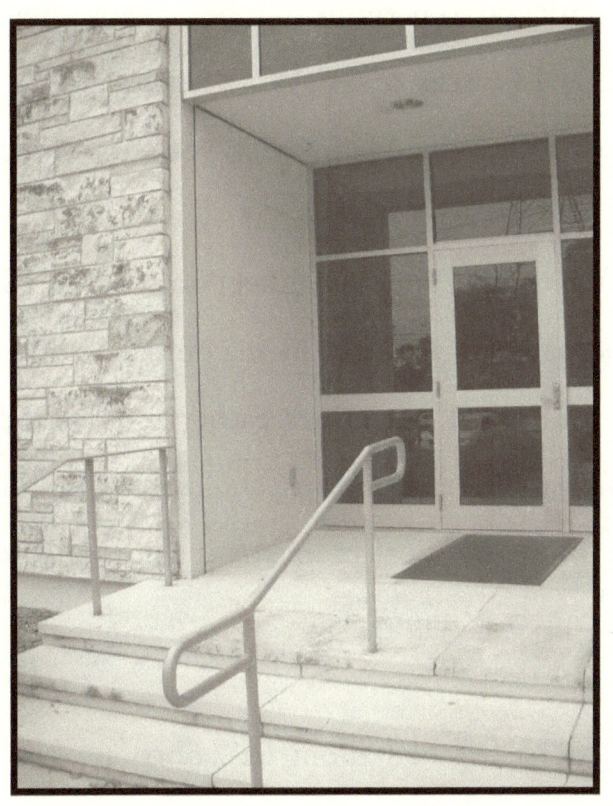

There's a secret behind this door that you're not supposed to know about: the baby is not the only one who dies --- YOU are being assaulted right along with your baby.

OK, let's get this right out in the open --- I've said the "B-word" twice now. You'll never hear the word "baby" behind this door. Here's what you will hear: "Product of conception", "contents of the uterus", It's not a baby until 14 weeks".

Let me ask you something --- if he's a baby after 14 weeks, what is he at 13 weeks & 6 days --- a puppy? ----a zucchini? News Flash: If he's not a baby, then you're not pregnant.

What's assaulting you? It's called Post-Abortion Syndrome, & it can actually kill you. If it doesn't physically kill you, it can make you wish it had. Migraines, eating disorders, relationship problems, inability to bond, psychological numbing, mood swings & more. Physical problems including increased risk for breast cancer & more.

"But I don't feel bad about my abortion" ---- you don't have to. Studies have shown that PAS may well be chemical.

Translation: It simply does not matter how you feel about abortion. You could see your abortion as the best thing that ever happened to you & you still will experience some form of PAS.

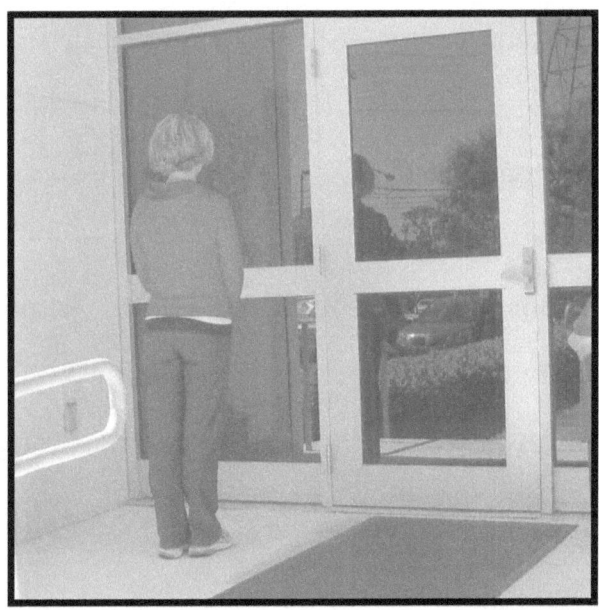

There's a woman standing outside this door. Why is she there? She's there because she's pregnant & she's decided that she cannot be pregnant.

Why? Because she's too young/too old. Because she can't afford to: raise a child, interrupt her career, her education, her life. Because her parents will be: disappointed, hurt, outraged.

Because her man will: leave her if he feels trapped, divorce her if he finds out she's cheated, assume the baby isn't his even if she hasn't cheated & leave her, want the baby & be hurt to find that she doesn't.

She's feeling totally alone &, although it hasn't even happened yet, she's feeling ---- empty. Above all, she just wants it to be OVER so that her life can get back to the way it was -- back to normal.

Three thousand three hundred women stand outside this door every day in the United States, for 3300 different, complex reasons, with 3300 different, complex combinations of feelings.

Who is she? She's your mother, your grandmother, your sister, your daughter, your aunt, your cousin, your niece, your friend, your co-worker, & maybe ---- she's you.

If you are a woman in the US today, & you have reached the age of 45, there is a 43% chance that you have had at least one abortion. That means ---

She's you, or someone that you know ---- or both.

EVERYONE who's reading these words right now knows someone who has had an abortion. Statistics say you know more than one person. I know, some of you are saying "Not me -- I don't know anyone" ---- there's only one reason you're saying that --- you just don't know who it is yet.

All of us have one very important thing in common:

Like the woman standing outside the door marked "Showers" at Auschwitz, we've all been lied to, & we all believed the lie.

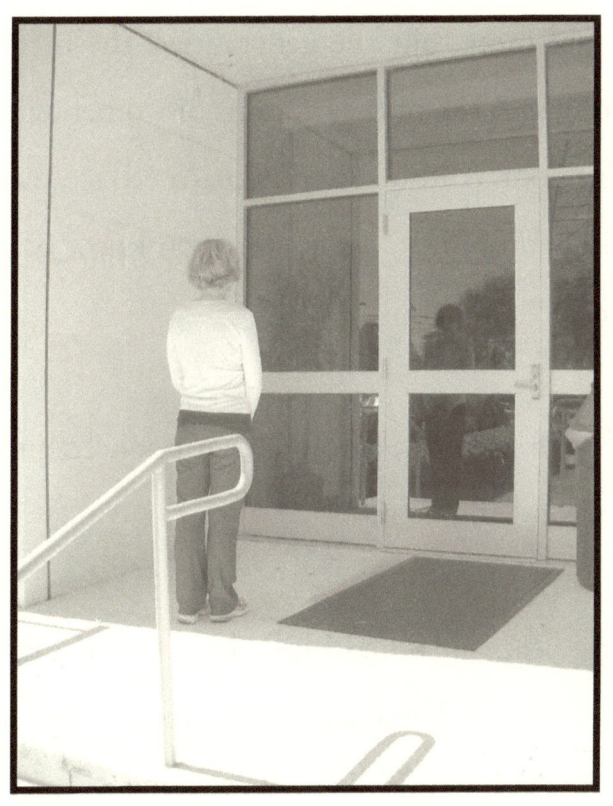

My Story

This book is a series of 6 stories. The first one is mine. It's first because it's the jumping off point for all the rest. Stories like the one you're about to hear begin 3300 times every single day, all across America.

Names have been changed, or left out. The specifics of this story are mine, but the generalities, the broad strokes, could belong to ANY of the millions of women who've stood outside this door. And if she could turn & face you now, her face would be familiar --- someone you know & love ------ maybe you.

Come with me now, through that door, & into the land that lies beyond abortion.

I was 34 years old when I killed my son. If I had allowed him to live, his due date would have been my 35th birthday. I was 21 weeks pregnant. I had felt movement.

Until 2 days before the abortion, I did not know I was pregnant. Doctors had always told me I couldn't conceive, & I had had 2 negative pregnancy tests. I thought I had a tumor. I thought I was dying--- then I found out.

I was in a very dysfunctional marriage. I was hiding -- behind alcohol & cocaine.

All of which made me the Poster Child for the so-called "Justifiable Abortion" . Any one of the conditions & circumstances I've just told you about is what the Abortion Industry (oh yes, it IS an industry) tells us is a good reason to "terminate the pregnancy" (read: "terminate the baby"). And that's exactly what I heard ---- from everyone.

From the "Dr" at the "Clinic" : "It'll probably have Fetal Alcohol Syndrome --maybe also cocaine addiction -- probably brain damage --- abort it".

Same "Dr": "Good thing you came in now -- one more week & we wouldn't be able to help you".

Friend #1: "You want to have kids, you just don't want to have them right now".

Friend #2: "Brain damage?? --- kinder to save it from that kind of life".

Minister: "Send it back to God".

Yep -- I was the Poster child for "Choice". In California, where Phil & I were living at the time, it was easy as pie. Just claim your husband's left you, & Medi-Cal pays for everything. Path of least resistance: Go ahead & do it.

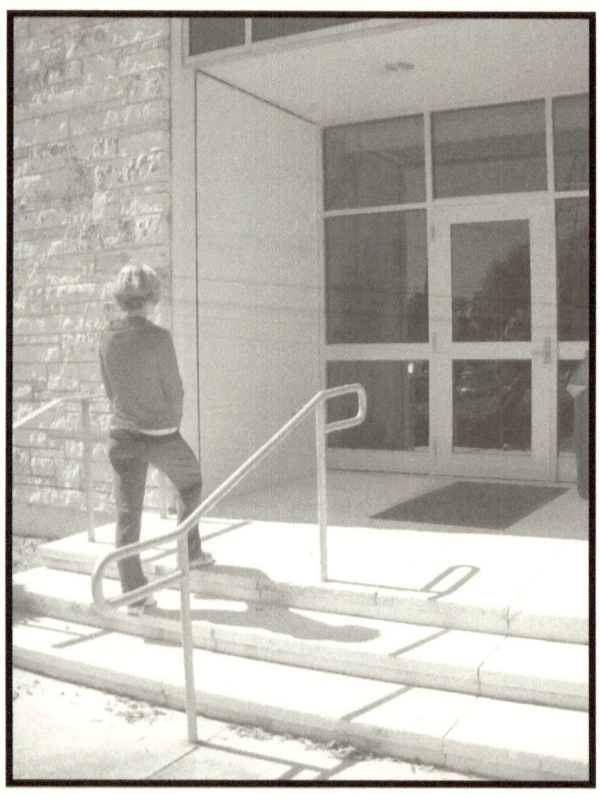

What follows is a series of snapshots --- I've blocked out most of the smaller details.

Drugs to dilate the cervix ---

Paying extra for general anesthesia (Medi-Cal didn't cover that)----

Counting backwards --- unconscious ---

Eyes closed, coming around, hearing a male & a female voice --- male: "Did I get it all?" --- female: "Yeah, it was a boy -- it's all here ---"

(sound of a curtain sliding on runners) "Oh, you're awake -- sit up slowly ---"

Tight shot of a giant pink stuffed rabbit in the corner (we'll come back to him later -- he's important).

Out to the car & Blinding sunlight ---

Dancing that night -- showing off my nice flat tummy ---

Like I said, I went ahead & did it -- like millions of my sisters before me, I believed the door marked "Showers" at Auschwitz really was a shower & I went in.

And that, according to the Abortion Industry, should be the end of the story. Here's the final paragraph as they would write it: "She made the often-difficult, decision to choose to terminate the pregnancy. Her life returned to normal, & she looked forward to having healthy, wanted children in the future" . --- She lived happily ever after.

Not one word of the paragraph above is true. It is pure, unadulterated bull----, & you're about to find out the Truth.

After the abortion, a really interesting thing happens: Mother Nature shows up --- BIG time. Mother Nature shows up in the form of the strongest natural instinct on the planet ------ the Maternal Instinct.

It's there in ALL of us who are female, whether we want it or not. I have many gay friends, & I assure you, it's there even in women who'd rather be men. It's there in all of us who have NO children. We take it out on animals, by making our pets our children. We take it out on other people's kids, on other adults, on inanimate objects --- but we DO take it out on someone or something, because it's in us until the day we die, & it MUST have an outlet.

It's there in the chemical bonding, the physical bonding process that starts right after conception, bonding mother to baby for life.

This instinct is stronger than the instinct to survive. We've all heard the countless stories of mothers sacrificing their own lives to save their children. Well, even though we've "chosen" to participate in the killing of our own baby, that deep, primal, physical hard-wiring is still there. In fact, the chemical bonding is still there even after the baby is NOT!

So, even though some of us (like me) go out dancing after the abortion, our bodies KNOW. Our bodies know that something, we're not quite sure what, but SOMETHING ---- is just not right.

That's when we experience what I've come to call "The Moment". The time frame varies as widely as the women who've walked through that door. Sometimes it's a day later, an hour, a week. Someone told me it happened to her in the little room where you put your clothes back on.

"The Moment" is not really a minute --- it can be just a few seconds, but it feels like hours. I'm going to attempt to show you what it's like:

In that Moment, all the warm-fuzzy nicknames you've called abortion dissolve away. Stark reality jumps up & hits you right between the eyes. Every cell in your body knows, really KNOWS, what you have done. There's a voice inside you & it's screaming: "I have just committed the most unnatural act -- I have just killed my own child --- Oh my God, what have I done?"

It is the scariest, most painful feeling you can imagine -- Like sticking your hand into fire & holding it there ------- EVERYTHING in you says "PULL BACK --- RUN AWAY ---- RUNRUNRUNRUNRUNRUN !!!!"

And that's exactly what we do. We run away. Some of us spend the rest of our lives running away from that Moment.

That escape route, that running away process, is what Post Abortion Syndrome (PAS) is all about. Ever wonder if there's really a Heaven & Hell? Well, I hope there's a Heaven, but I don't know for sure. As for Hell --- I can tell you from experience that Hell is absolutely real, & it's called PAS.

But what if we COULD just run away? ---- bury that awful few seconds of KNOWING under layers & layers of concrete, like Jimmy Hoffa under an off-ramp somewhere, forever hidden & forgotten. Brush it permanently under the rug & never think about it again --- sounds pretty good, doesn't it --- that would almost make it OK --- almost get us off the hook.

But we can't.

And the reason that we can't is that we have a DEAD BABY. ---- no less than the mother whose child died in any other way.

----- The fact that we participated in the killing

doesn't make the baby any less dead !!

Think about this: What happens when a woman has a baby who dies in his crib of some awful infant disease or Sudden Infant Death Syndrome --- what do we do as a society? We all feel her pain, don't we?

"Oh poor Mary, her baby died" -- we have grieving & mourning, we have a funeral, a tiny casket ,a graveside ceremony, a small headstone, a gathering of friends & family afterward at the house or the Hall. --- We have everything that goes with the death/grieving/mourning process --- because that's what it's all about, isn't it? --It's not for the dead person, it's for US, the living, to help us deal with the fact that someone has died & move on with our lives.

Well, the Post-Abortive mother has a dead baby too (remember, the fact that she participated in the killing doesn't make the baby any less dead) ---- what does our society say to her? ---- we say

"Baby?? ---- What baby??"

Lets stop for a minute & consider this. She not only has a very real dead child who she can't grieve & mourn for (she thinks she doesn't deserve to anyhow, since she participated in killing him) --- she has a very real dead child that Society won't even allow her to acknowledge EVER EXISTED IN THE FIRST PLACE !!!!

Now, if you know anything about psychology, (& I've learned a lot about it, having 2 friends who are Psychiatrists), you know that when someone close to you dies, you MUST grieve & mourn that death.

If you are somehow prevented from going through the normal, healthy grieving process, you are in serious, serious psychological trouble. They call it Impacted Grief. There are people in institutions because of Impacted Grief & complications that arise from it.

The Post-Abortive woman is experiencing Impacted Grief, Survivor-Guilt, & a whole spectrum of other problems, all under the huge umbrella of Post-Abortion Syndrome.

What are the symptoms? ---- Ready? --- Migraines, eating disorders, relationship problems, inability to bond, psychological numbing, mild to severe depression, radical, bi-polar type mood swings, dissociation, & we haven't even scratched the surface --- these are just some of the emotional symptoms. Then there are the physical problems including increased risk of breast cancer.

How do you know if someone is Post-Abortive? Impossible to tell. We cover the whole spectrum. We range from the Compulsive Perfectionist -- I have a good friend I call Super Woman who's a perfect example of this end of the spectrum: She had her abortion 20 years ago so she could stay in grad school & get her PhD. Now, 20 years later, she has the perfect house, perfect husband, perfect career, perfect children. She's driven. We'll meet her again a little further along in this journey -----

From the Compulsive Perfectionist like Super Woman, all the way down to the other end of the spectrum --- the Compulsively Self-Destructive. That was me.

I divorced my first husband and entered into an equally dysfunctional second marriage. I continued to hide behind alcohol and cocaine, but never so it showed --- I functioned in

the world of Intangible Sales (admissions at private colleges &
modeling schools). Ironic, huh ---- I was a dream-merchant,
& quite good at it too.

At every crucial point in my life or career, I managed to
shoot myself in the foot. I sabotaged every aspect of my life.
Subtle, & not-so-subtle self-destructive behavior is typical of
a Post Abortive woman at this end of the scale.

My 2 Psychiatrist friends have taught me that the way
you see your Self, your deep-down Self-Image affects the way
you relate to everything, & most important, EVERYONE
around you.

So, you see PAS doesn't just affect the woman --- it touches
her husband, her partner, her children, her family, her friends,
her co-workers --- EVERYONE she relates to every day. Like
the rock thrown into water --- the rock disappears, but the
ripples go on ----- into infinity.

These next few words may save yours or someone else's life,
so listen: THERE'S A WAY OUT !!!

It's a process, much like a 12-step program, but much less structured, & very adjustable to the individual person. Keep reading -- you'll find out about many, many ways to access the healing process later.

I found out about it almost by accident -- or so I thought at the time (I don't believe in "accidents" or "coincidences" any more). Here's what happened:

After 13 years in California, I moved back to the East Coast where I was raised. A friend of mine took me into an Orthodox Christian church -- it was the first time I'd ever been in one. ---- now don't get all nervous here --- this isn't going to turn into a preachy book --- trust me.

Remember, I'd spent the last 13 years in CA, where they have the ever-popular Religion-of-the-Month club. In my politically-correct quest to be "spiritual", like a good Californian, I had dabbled in EVERYTHING --- Hinduism, Buddhism, Roman Catholicism, Judaism, Tao, Islam, Wicca, Santa Ria --- you name it, I had studied it. If there was a temple or an ashram or a mud hut you could go into to worship anything, I had been there --- but never an Orthodox church.

My friend insisted I go, & it was like a movie scene --- I was awe-struck. There was this feeling that this was where I was supposed to be. Started taking classes, & 6 months later, I was ready to be inducted into the Church.

As part of this process, you need to go to confession. I'd studied Catholicism, but I'd never actually been to confession, so I asked Father what the procedure was.

He said "Make a list of all your sins" --- uh-oh. You know what my life had been like up to that point --- where to even start? --- But I was game if he was, "OK Father -- how many days do these things take & where do you sleep?"

The man has patience. He said "Why don't you just make an outline --- you know -- general categories ---". So I did. I had almost finished my confession, when I tacked on, as a complete afterthought, "Oh, & I had this abortion a few years ago --------" Dead silence.

A few embarrassing seconds passed, & I looked over at Father (we were in his office, not a Confessional, so I could see him), who was quietly crying. I said "Father, why are you crying?" --- he looked at me & said "I'm crying for your baby".

The room disappeared

I wasn't sitting in a chair in an office, I was sitting up slowly on a gurney, & in front of me was ---- a giant pink stuffed rabbit ------. That Moment, that horrible, sticking-your-hand-into-fire Moment ---- that I thought was totally buried ---- came raging back, multiplied by a thousand.

I slid out of the chair onto the floor --- I was crying --- great racking sobs, & I didn't stop for about an hour.

My 2 psychiatrist friends tell me that, at that moment, I experienced a great psychological breakthrough --- I came out of my denial about my dead child. I also have 2 Baptist friends who are equally certain that, at that moment, I was saved. I think all 4 of them are right, & it's probably both.

Whatever you want to call it, I'm grateful that it happened because, although I didn't know it at the time, that's the day my healing process actually began.

On the way home, I started to get angry. I'm not talking "Oh-darn-it" angry, I'm talking pounding-on-the-steering-wheel angry.

Wait a damn minute --- maybe there's a NAME for this Thing that just knocked me out of my chair --- maybe there's a NAME for this Thing that's been ruining my life for the past 16 years.

Went straight to the library (remember, this is 1997--- not everybody had computers at home), & did some research ---- actually, a LOT of research.

Note: Right here, you may want to put the book down, & go get yourself a nice cup of something before you continue reading. Trust me. You're going to be surprised, & quite possibly angry, at what you're about to see.

Here's what I found out: I was NOT alone & I was NOT crazy. Indeed, there WAS a name for it --- it was called Post-Abortion Syndrome. And here's what disturbed me the most--- there had been NINE books written, & there were TWENTY-ONE national organizations just for people like me, women (& men -- yes, men too) with PAS. ---- remember, this is 1997 -- there are many more today.

Think about that for a minute: This Thing had affected every aspect of my life for over a decade, & had come close to killing me -----

AND I HAD NEVER EVEN HEARD ABOUT IT !!!!

I'll bet that right now, unless you're really familiar with all or this, that you can't name even one of those books or one of those big, national organizations.

Know WHY you don't even know they exist ---? Because the Abortion Industry, with its deep pockets, & big advertising money, doesn't WANT you to know.

If you knew that there are many many books & many many big, national organizations with websites & resources all to help people with PAS --- if you knew all that, why then you'd also know the Dirty Little Secret behind that door called "Choice":

The baby is NOT the only one who dies.

Big parts of his mother die right along with him.

And she keeps right on dying -- emotionally, spiritually, psychologically, & sometimes physically (yes, some of us commit suicide) UNTIL something either shakes her out of her denial, & she begins the healing process (as happened to me), OR -----

She takes her PAS to her grave ---- never connecting the dots --- never realizing that her migraines, her eating disorders, her relationship problems, her inability to bond, all the things that have been ruining her life ----- all stem back to something that she may have done 10, 20, 30, or even 40 years ago. ---- Something that she THINKS she feels perfectly OK about now ----

Way back in the beginning of this book, I told you a statistic. Well, turn up the volume, here it comes:

If you are a woman, who has reached the age of 45 in the USA today, there is a 43% chance that you have had at least one abortion.

Look around you ---- I'm everywhere --- WE'RE everywhere. We surround you every day of your life. I'm your mother, your grandmother, your sister, your daughter, your wife, your aunt your cousin, you friend, your teacher, your student, your co-worker --- & maybe ---- I'm you.

You KNOW someone who has had an abortion. Statistics say you know more than one of us. If you're thinking that you don't, there's only one reason: you don't know who it is yet.

There's a famous video, made by a man I'm honored to know, Dr. Bernard Nathanson, called "The Silent Scream" -- you can't hear the baby screaming as he dies in an abortion. Well, we are Post-Abortive mothers, & we're in agony too, only we're not just silent -- we're invisible --- & some of us are REALLY invisible because we SEEM to be doing so well.

Remember my friend, the compulsive perfectionist I call Super Woman? If you ask her today, how she feels about her abortion, that she had 20 years ago so she could stay in grad school, I know exactly what she'll say --- I've heard it many times: "OH yes, very difficult decision, regrettable & very difficult. But, look at my life --- I made the right choice".

And, if you look at her life today, it looks pretty darn perfect. She & her husband are both at the top of their careers, they live in a mansion, both make more money than they can spend. They have 2 kids in High School --- both over-achievers. The girl, a freshman, could be a model & is a straight-A student. The boy, a senior, also straight-A's, is a star athlete, & has his choice of Ivy League schools. Super Woman & her husband belong to all the right clubs & are sought-after A-listers.

Sure enough, looking at all that wealth & success, it looks like she's right.

Let's take a peek behind the movie set scenery now, shall we? Her husband, Mr. Perfect, is cheating on her & sleeping with everything that moves. She knows it --- she's in denial about that too. Her son, Mr. Most Likely to Succeed, has, along with all his trophies, a very expensive cocaine habit, & his sister is being treated for bulimia --- none of this is a secret to Superwoman. She has her own problem -- 2 or 3 times a month, she gets the kind of debilitating migraines where you throw up every half hour. ----- not all that perfect, is it?

Denying that she's in that prison will not make the bars melt away.

In my travels around the country, I often hear these words: "You're right, I DO know someone who's had an abortion. Maybe she's in denial, but she seems to be just fine --- why dredge up all that pain if we don't have to?"

First of all, she's not fine. She may be in pain on some whole other level, & it may involve a part of her life that SEEMS totally unrelated. --- More important, many say that PAS may well be largely chemical ---- and if that's true, the way she feels (or does NOT feel) about her abortion SIMPLY DOES NOT MATTER !!

In other words, she could see abortion as the best thing that ever happened to mankind, & she will STILL experience some form of PAS. It is literally her own body not allowing her to forget what happened. It is PHYSICALLY impossible for a woman to forget a child she's lost.

One of the steps in the healing process is to name the baby who has died, & to finally grieve & mourn that death. Now I know that sounds morbid, but it's not at all. It's a very healthy, very necessary thing that we need to do to heal.

My son's name is Gabriel. If I had allowed him to live, he would have been 28 years old this past August 3rd.

About a year after my healing process began, I was watching a young mother carrying a baby boy about a year old through a church hall. She had him up on one hip, the way you carry kids that size, & she walked a little too close to the door & he hit his head.

After 2 or 3 stunned seconds, he opened his mouth, & began to shriek, as only a one year old can. You all know what I mean. Fire alarms have a lower decibel level.

She stood him on his feet, knelt down in front of him, & began rubbing his head, crooning over & over "Oh Mommy's so sorry you hurt your head---" . Amazing. Like turning off alight switch --- the shrieking stopped --- no more tears --- just like that ---- she had made it all better.

I thought nothing of it at the time, but it had resonated somewhere in my subconscious.

About 8 hours later, I found myself on my living room floor on my knees --- sobbing-- rocking back & forth & talking to my son, saying --- "Gabriel, Mommy is sorry ---- Mommy is so sorry ------"

There are no words for how that feels. At that moment, I would have given my life to reverse my "choice" & to let my baby live.

I'm glad that it happened, because it's a necessary part of my personal healing process. But it's also one of the reasons I began speaking out about PAS.

I speak out now for the millions of Post-Abortive mothers ---- my sisters, who, like me 14 years ago, have never heard of PAS --- who haven't connected any dots --- who only know that something's WRONG & it hurts.

I speak out now for the millions more, the family & friends who love us & who want to help, but don't know how.

But most of all, I speak about my experience so that neither you, nor anyone you care about will ever have to live through a moment like this one because you'll never have to heal from something like what I did to my son -----

AND TO MYSELF.

Read that last sentence again. It's important ---- "what I did to my son ---- AND TO MYSELF !!!

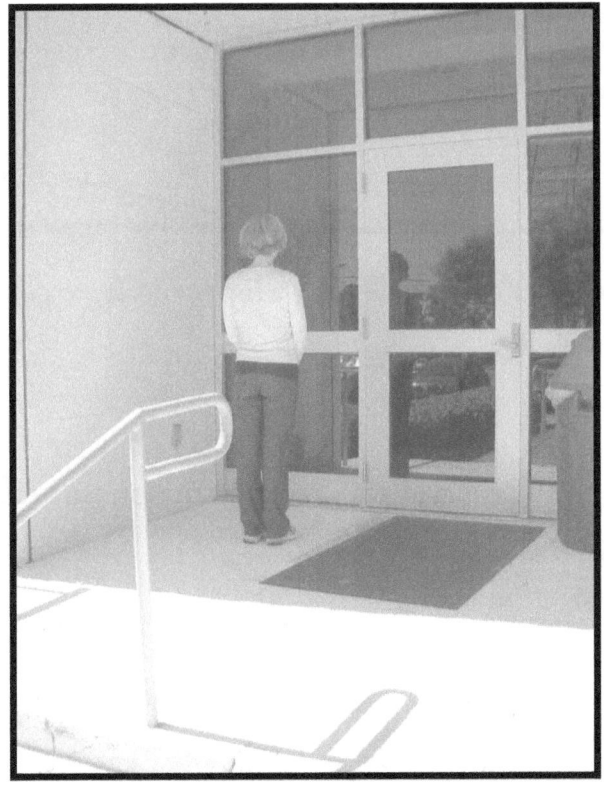

Abortion doesn't just kill your baby --- It hurts YOU.

When you "Choose" abortion, you are hurting YOURSELF.

OK, lets talk about that Self. Who are you, anyhow? You are unique among all other humans. Your special, individual

DNA is what makes you different from every other person on the planet.

Your DNA is undeniable, conclusive evidence & can identify you as the only person who could have committed a crime. ---- it is what makes you --- You.

And it is THERE at the moment of conception.

You were YOU at the moment of conception --- not some vague, potential you, but YOU -- the same person that you are today, in a much smaller body. --- Exactly the same as looking at a photo of yourself at the age of 2 -- still you, just much smaller than you are today.

Your DNA was there, in that moment that the sperm & the egg, incomplete apart, became complete when joined together, & there YOU were. For the next 9 months or so, that one cell divided & divided countless times, you grew, you sucked your thumb, you heard your mother's voice, & then, when it was time, you emerged from your mother's body ---- happy birthday.

And just think --- it all started some 40 weeks ago, when YOU were that one little cell -- my how you've grown.

"A person's a person, no matter how small".

But what if your mother had made a different "Choice"? --- Even if she had walked through that door just a few hours after conception, she would have been destroying, killing YOU --- no less than if she had killed the 2 year old in the photo --- you, in a much smaller body.

If your mom is still living, maybe you should call her & say thanks.

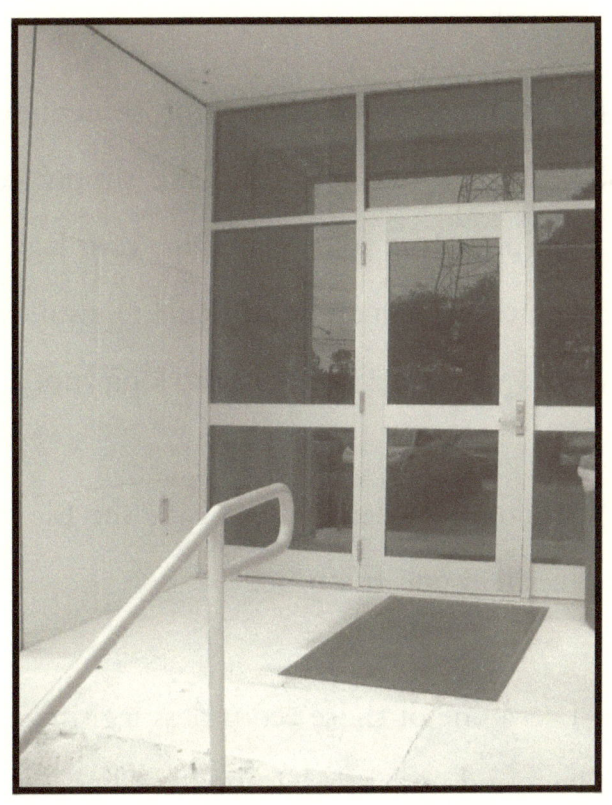

The Big Lie

Ok, now let's explore some of the lies you've been told by our politically-correct culture for your whole life.

The Big, Overriding Concept:

Abortion is a necessary choice for someone who, for countless, legitimate reasons, feels she simply cannot be pregnant right now. It is your Way Out, your legal right, & like some medicines, it may be difficult to swallow, but it's good for you & you'll feel better in the long run.

There are actually 3 deadly lies inside the Big Lie above. Let's examine them one at a time.

LIE #1 --- Every one of those "countless legitimate reasons" can be found under this umbrella: Choose abortion so that your life will not have to change. (read: you can stay in school, keep your man, keep your career, stay on the team, keep supporting your family, etc. etc.) After the abortion, your life will return to normal.

TRUTH #1 ---

It's exactly the opposite --- From the moment your baby dies, your life CHANGES & is never the same. The physical process that bonds you to your baby starts at conception, & stays there even after the baby is gone. No matter how deeply you bury it, YOUR OWN BODY KNOWS that something is very wrong.

LIE #2 --- It's your Way Out, your legal right. (in other words, it's right up there with your right to vote. Women before you have sacrificed & fought for these rights. "It's my body, & my right to choose"

TRUTH #2 ---

LOTS of things that are legal can, & will hurt you --- & may even kill you. Let's look at some of them: (legal-age) DRINKING, (licensed) DRIVING, (legal-age) SMOKING (prescription) DRUGS. All of these are perfectly legal, but is there an adult in the civilized world today who doesn't know that every one of the perfectly legal activities above can hurt you & can even kill you?

The best example is smoking. I'm old enough to remember when smoking was advertised EVERYWHERE--- on TV, on billboards, on buses & subways. I'll bet some of you can even remember the Marlboro Man, or Joe Camel, or Virginia Slims ads. Smoking was Everywhere. It was glamorous, sophisticated, a rite of passage. Celebrities endorsed cigarette brands. Ads told us to have a cigarette after dinner instead of dessert.

You could smoke Anywhere -- at work, in ALL restaurants & bars, some movie theaters, on planes, on trains, pretty much anywhere.

We learned from our beloved movie stars that a cigarette could be many things: It was a prop used to make gestures more emphatic, it was a device to buy time (the long, slow lighting up), it was a romance-starter ("light?"), it was a romance-ender (the contemptuous grinding out), it was Masculinity (James Dean & the ever-present cigarette) it was Female Glamour (the long black cigarette holder). It was all things to all people in all situations.

And best of all -- remember "You've come a long way Baby!" ----?? For those of you who don't --- Virginia Slims cigarettes became one of the icons of the Feminist Movement with their famous ads. Every ad had the same theme: An "old" sepia-toned picture was shown of a woman in the 19th century being denied access to a men's club, being booted out of contention for a job, or just generally being relegated to the pink-collar ghetto just for being a woman.

Then, right next to that picture, we saw a glorious full-color picture of the same woman, in modern dress doing something daring, glamorous or innovative usually while smoking a Virginia Slims.

"You've Come a Long Way, Baby" became one of the most effective marketing tools of the day --- & lots of cool, sophisticated, glamorous young women began a habit that would last for life.

Then came lung cancer ---- the horrifying specter of undeniable facts & statistics --- the toothpaste was out of the tube, & try as they might, the tobacco industry couldn't push it back in --- SMOKING COULD KILL YOU !! -- All of a sudden, everything changed. No more Marlboro Man, no more Joe Camel, no more romantic smoking scenes in movies, & of course, "You've Come a Long Way, Baby" went the way of the 8 track tape player.

America woke up. I love my country. Once we Americans are shown the undeniable Truth about something, there is no turning back. A line from one of my favorite novels reads: "It has happened, he is awake. Now it will be like holding unbroken horses."

Abortion is just as legal as smoking -- more so. Cigarettes have a warning label, abortion mills do not ----yet.

LIE #3 --- "Like some medicines, it may be difficult to swallow, but it's good for you, & you'll feel better in the long run." --- Another common way to put it: "It's just like having your tonsils out -- a minor surgical procedure that gets rid of an unnecessary piece of tissue. You have your tonsils out, you go home, & you feel better. Abortion is a minor detour -- a small necessary procedure, like getting your tonsils out, so you can eliminate the problem & get on with your life" ---- this may be the cruelest lie of all. ("It's just a shower")

TRUTH #3 ---

From the moment the sperm & the egg unite YOUR body is changing. Think about what happens over that 9 months. Your baby is growing at warp speed starting with the second he's conceived. YOUR body is changing -- your body is beginning to bond with your baby. Let's examine that bond for a minute.

Psychologists have called your mother "your first love" ---- the bond between mother & child lasts forever. During extreme stress, when we believe ourselves to be near death, 99 out of 100 people will call out for their mother.

Soldiers, dying on the battlefield call out for Mama. And the converse is also true --- we've all heard the stories of mothers somehow knowing when their child, who's thousands of miles away is in danger.

That hard-wired bonding begins in the female body at the moment of conception. We who are female all have that fierce, primal instinct whether we want it or not. Abortion takes all of Nature & turns it upside down.

It takes a perfectly normal female human being who, if left to Nature, would DIE to protect her child, & compels her to KILL that child. IT MIGHT AS WELL TELL HER TO HACK OFF HER OWN ARM. ----- And it gets worse. The Abortion Industry & our politically-correct culture says, that while hacking off your own arm is slightly unpleasant, it's perfectly normal, & you'll feel much better afterward.

This is, I think, the essence of PAS. Before she's walked through that door, when her child is still alive inside her, & that deep primal bond is already forming, there is a Voice. There is a timeless Knowing deep within that This Is Wrong. We stifle it, we drown it out, we lock it in a soundproof room, but like a deep underground stream, it is There.

Her mind says "You made the right choice, now get on with your life". She tells everyone "I feel fine about it -- difficult choice, but I did the only thing I could do & I've moved on".

Her own body knows the truth. It happens at the oddest times --- watching childbirth on TV, walking through the infant dept. -- it can hit her like a punch in the stomach or just the faint echo of a Voice -- not quite heard, but There.

Her body is screaming "Someone killed my baby" --- & all that rage has to have somewhere to go -- she can't let it out, because that would mean acknowledging that Something Is Wrong. ---- so all that rage turns inward & begins to devour her. It starts. The migraines, the eating disorders, the relationship problems, the inability to bond, & on & on & on.

And it doesn't stop there. Your deep-down Self-Image affects the way you relate to Everyone so even if you planned on being stoic & bearing the burden of PAS all by yourself, you can't. Everyone who's close to you is going to bear that burden right along with you & you can't avoid it.

Like a cold, damp fog, PAS permeates & colors every relationship --- husband, children, family, friends, --- the cancer spreads. --- So you see, it's not just you.

OK, so now you know --- the toothpaste is out of the tube, & there's no pushing it back in. What are you going to do? ---- Before you say anything, let's go on to our next story.

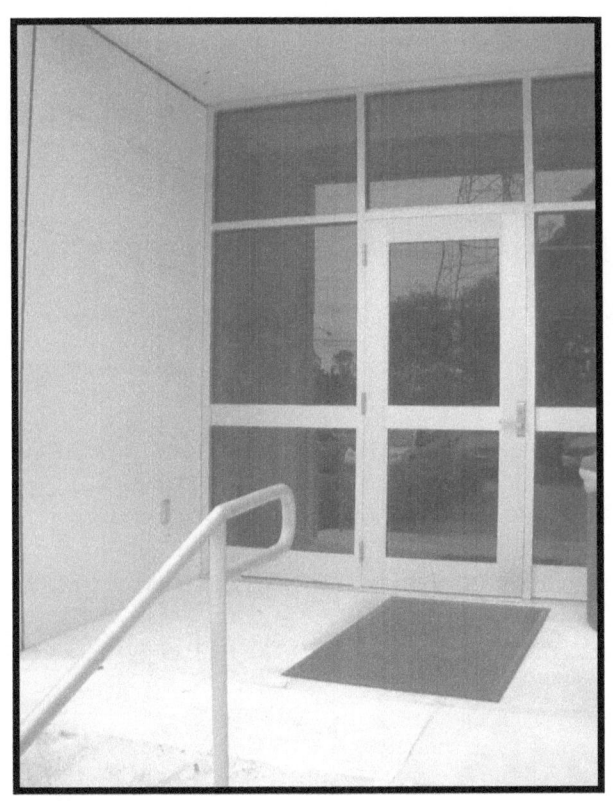

LACI'S STORY

I have 4 words for you: Laci Peterson, Conner Peterson. For those who don't remember, I'm talking about the famous Laci Peterson murder case that happened a few years ago in California.

Laci Peterson was a young wife & soon-to-be mother in CA who went missing when she was 8 or 9 months pregnant & due to give birth any day. Laci & her husband, Scott knew the baby was a boy, & they'd chosen to name him Conner. Laci was happy & excited about having her first child & the nursery was all ready --- then suddenly -- Laci was gone.

I'll spare you the smarmy details. Scott spent weeks doing a bad job of acting the concerned husband. Then Laci & Conner's bodies were found. Scott Peterson was tried & found guilty of murdering TWO people -- his wife Laci AND his son Conner.

The Unborn Victims of Violence Act came to be known as "Laci & Conner's Law". Put simply, it says that, if I'm pregnant & you kill me, you have killed TWO people. HOW pregnant? --- the old joke comes to mind here, about the girl who was "only a little bit pregnant" -----. In most states, the law just says "pregnant" --- in some states, it stipulates that I must be a certain number of weeks (14,12, 8 , etc,) pregnant.

Now that's silly, isn't it ??? Let's take the state that stipulates 8 weeks for example ---- What if Scott had killed Laci when she was 7 weeks & 6 days pregnant? --- is the baby not Conner? Has Scott killed a puppy? --- of course not ---- He has killed his son Conner Peterson.

This case & Laci & Conner's story is important for another reason --- it's important because of the media. All through the trial, Conner was called Conner (not "the fetus" or "the unborn child"). When doctors testified about what happens to a baby who is still inside his mother when she dies, a whole nation was moved.

Conner was a real baby to us --- not some vague concept on a development chart, but a real baby who could FEEL PAIN ---

And then of course there were all the forensics people talking about DNA. Conner's DNA was there at conception, so even if Scott Peterson had committed his horrible crime when Laci was only a few days pregnant, he still would have killed TWO people. ---- Conner was Conner, & no one else from the moment he was conceived.

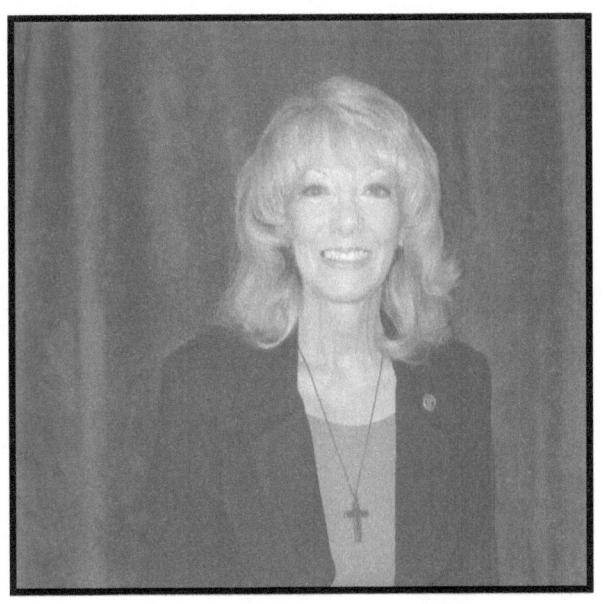

The Troublemaker

So when is a baby a baby? --- which brings me to our next story ---- the Troublemaker.

This happened very early in my life as a public speaker -- about 12 years ago.

They warned me about him. They said he was a "troublemaker". Big High School in New Jersey --- I was being paid to speak to all the juniors & seniors at a huge joint assembly. The principal & 2 teachers took me aside & pointed him out. Always asking speakers difficult or embarrassing questions --- don't call on him --.

Now I'm a teacher's kid. My mom taught High School for 42 years, so when teachers give me that kind of tip, I tend to listen, because they usually know what (& who) they're talking about.

I finished my presentation in the big auditorium. The question & answer session had gone really well. I'd brought lots of the visual aids that teens like & the kids were both fascinated & respectful.

I looked at the big clock in the back & there were easily 5 more minutes before the bell. One hand was still up & waving enthusiastically ---- yep --- it was him.

I looked over at one of the teachers & she was almost imperceptibly shaking her head, as was the principal.

I've been in these situations before. ---- Easy. You just say "Hold your question for a minute while I clarify this" --- &

you go into a long elaboration on the previous answer. Then when the bell rings, you invite the person to come up & ask his question individually ---- Easy.

At least it SHOULD have been. But the Q & A had gone so well -- & this was just a cute little boy (15 or 16, small for his age, with red hair & freckles). After all, I was a professional speaker -- I'd been heckled by 50 year old intellectuals -- what could this cute little kid do ?

I put on my best Earth Mother smile, & said "OK, what's your question?"

He stood up. Bad sign. None of the others had stood. He drew himself up to his full height of maybe 5 foot 4, & said "I'm Catholic -- I know it's a baby right from conception, but when does the Law say it's a baby?" --- Triumphant grin firmly in place, he sat down, folded his arms, & waited.

In my head, I was having a talk with God --- actually I was yelling at God --- "OK, You got me into this, now You get me out".

Then it happened. I opened my mouth, & the words came out --- "Good question! -- whether a baby is a baby depends entirely on the lady he's inside of."

"Let's say she's been confirmed to be 11 weeks pregnant, OK? -- 1ˢᵗ Scenario: She wants him. She's happy & excited to be pregnant & here's what happens: we have baby showers & grandparents make toasts at dinner, & NAMES are chosen & sonogram pictures are shown around.

And what is HE doing at 11 weeks? -- He's sucking his thumb, making a fist, & kicking -- he can feel heat, touch, light & hear noise -- he's had brain waves for weeks now -- wonder what he's thinking ---

It's a big deal & a big celebration. Her responsibility to him as his mom is to protect him & love him & make sure he's healthy for the whole 9 months that he's inside her.------- Baby showers, names chosen, celebrations -- HE'S A BABY!

2ⁿᵈ Scenario: Same woman, same 11 weeks pregnant, same baby. This time, she is not happy to be pregnant & she does not want him. Here's what happens: our Politically-Correct culture says that this VERY SAME BABY is NOT a baby at all -- he is an extra piece of tissue & she has the same responsibility to him as she has to the hamburger she had for lunch. She eliminates him from her body & from life."

Long seconds went by. Off to my left, one of the teachers was dabbing at her eyes.

The Troublemaker looked different. It was the look we all get for one small moment, usually when we're very young, when we see something really, truly Wrong for the first time. Red-faced & scowling, forgetting to raise his hand, he shouted "But that's not RIGHT!"

I wanted to hug him. Sometimes I think the Young see injustice in sharper focus than we elders do. The Troublemaker was Everyman at that moment. He was Righteous Indignation itself. The other students, underneath their armor of suave teenage sophistication, all understood ----- they all GOT IT. The world hadn't had time to smooth out their edges & put the blinders on their sense of injustice ---- yet. Irrationally, I hoped it never would.

That day happened 12 years ago. In my travels, I've mentioned the boy's question & the answer many times. Afterward, I often hear compliments on what a great answer it was. I smile & say thank you.

Unless the person I'm talking to is a priest or a minister --- then I say what they, as clergy, already know: when the Troublemaker asked his question, I spoke the words, but it wasn't I who answered.

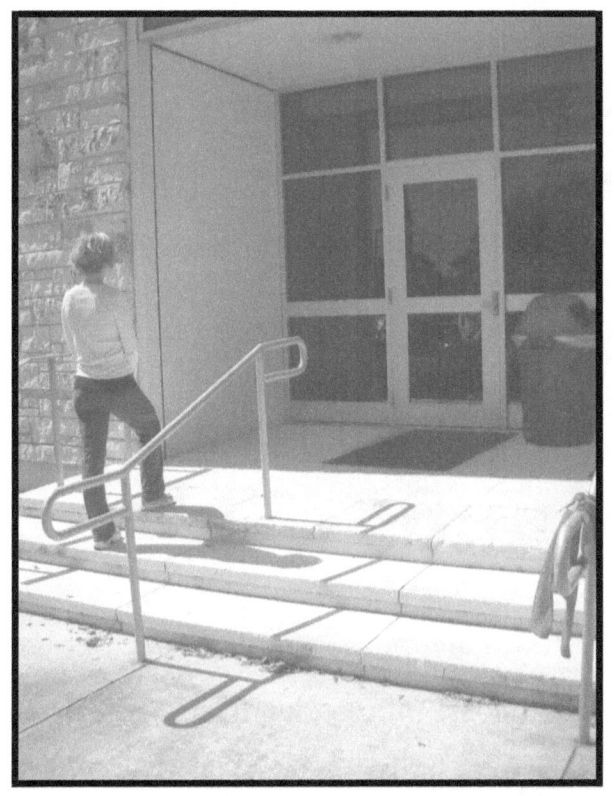

GIANNA

But what if the baby is not wanted, the mother has an abortion, & oops ---- the baby is born ALIVE?? Now that's a tricky one, isn't it?

The mother's intention, & the "Dr.'s" intention was to abort --- but here we have a live baby --- alive outside his mother's body --- this wasn't supposed to happen.

Which brings us to the story of Gianna.

Back in 2003, I shared a stage in Rhode Island with someone I'll never forget. I doubt that anyone who's ever seen her ever forgets her.

As sometimes happens, the organizers were running around arranging last minute details for the event which was being held in a huge hall. I knew that my half of the day was to be after lunch, from 1:00 PM to 4, & the other person they'd hired was to have the 9:00 AM to noon spot.

I hadn't seen any of the flyers promoting the event, & as for my fellow presenter, the person I was to share the event with , I knew her name, but nothing more.

I decided to attend the morning session & do something I rarely get a chance to do --- sit back & enjoy someone else's presentation & see what I could learn. I settled down in my front row seat. The MC made all the usual welcoming remarks to the crowd of several hundred people. Then he said "Now ladies & gentlemen, please welcome --- Gianna Jessen".

A pretty young woman slowly climbed the few stairs to the stage. I noticed she walked with a slight limp. She took the mike, sat down on a high stool, & began to sing.

Two things struck me right away. First, she wasn't just a pretty young woman --- she was truly beautiful. And second, she had an amazing voice --- the kind of voice that goes right through you from the first sound.

I was congratulating myself on my decision to be an audience member for the morning session, thinking I was about to enjoy a lot of great music. She finished her song to thunderous applause, but, rather than launching into another one, she began to speak instead.

Gianna Jessen began to tell her story.

(Here is a synopsis of what I heard that day)

She walks with a slight limp, a result of what she calls the "gift" of Cerebral Palsy. At birth, the doctors said she would never be able to hold her head up, sit up, crawl, or walk. Today she is a Christian singer & song writer & speaker & ---- Ready? ----- marathon runner !!

She shouldn't be running --- she shouldn't be even walking, & most miraculous of all ---- she shouldn't even be alive.

Gianna's biological mother was 17 when she had a saline abortion in her third trimester. After being burned alive for approximately 18 hours in the womb from the saline solution, Gianna was delivered alive in a Los Angeles County abortion clinic. Her medical records state: "Born during saline abortion" --- this is what caused her Cerebral Palsy. (you can read Gianna's entire biography on her website: giannajessen. com)

Having finished her story, this amazing woman then calmly launched into another beautiful original song. The standing ovation was the longest I've ever seen, before or since.

The Born-Alive Infants Protection Law says simply that, if a baby is born alive during an abortion, that baby should not be left to die.

You've just heard Gianna Jessen's story. Amazingly enough, there are actually some politicians living today who would DENY life support to a baby who, like Gianna, is born alive.

What do YOU think?

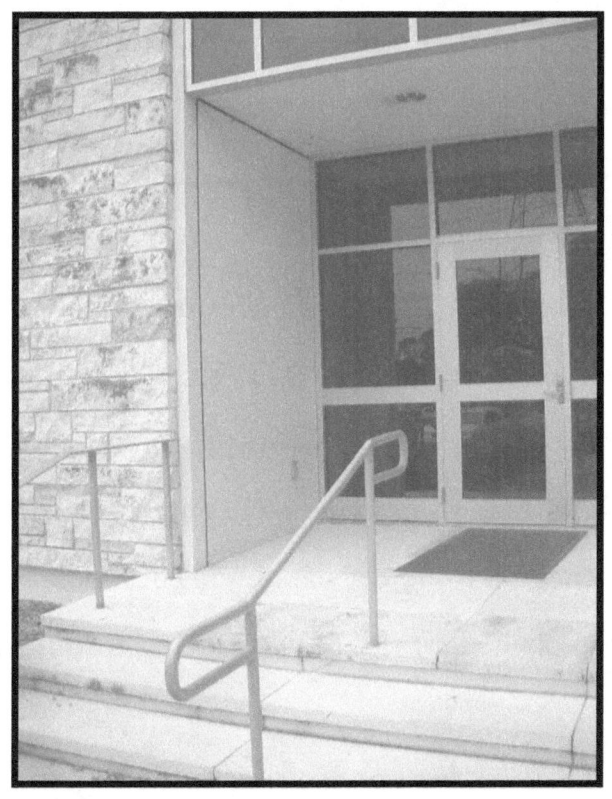

THE STORY OF MS. PC

Way back at the beginning of this book, I said you would hear a series of 6 stories. You're about to hear #5 --- the story of Ms. PC. ---- In a few minutes, you'll understand why I've given her that name.

It happened in a big auditorium on the West Coast--- one of the larger venues, it sat 1200 --- I had just finished my presentation of "Through the looking Glass, the Land Beyond Abortion".

There were the usual people coming up to the stage for handshakes, pictures, hugs, & CD's etc. ---- This went on for a few minutes,&, as the crowd was thinning out, I noticed an attractive 40-ish woman with an equally attractive teenage girl who appeared to be her daughter. They were standing at the very top of the first tier & not moving toward the stage.

I looked away & kept on shaking hands & getting pictures taken. After a few minutes, I was packing up to leave & meet the driver to go back to my hotel. I looked up, & they were still standing there.

The mother looked both ways to make sure they were the last ones there & came toward me, her daughter close behind.

None of this surprised me. There are often people (both male & female) who want to ask a question or share something with me in private after hearing a presentation. I put on my best benign, non-threatening face.

Mom speeded up as she saw me look up at her, --- her high heels clicking on the tile near the stage. I saw that this wasn't going to be the usual Q&A --- this woman was angry.

She halted about a foot from me.

"My daughter dragged me here to see you. She saw you yesterday at _____ High School." (THAT'S why the teen looked familiar --- I remembered her now -- she had come up to me afterward & given me a big high-five).

"I'm Pro-Choice. I've always been Pro-Choice --- & you have NOT changed my mind -- I'm still Pro-Choice." So, I was thinking to myself, why are you standing here now? --You didn't wait all this time just to tell me that.

"I want to know WHY I never heard about PAS before! This is AWFUL--- someone should be sued or put in jail for not bringing this out sooner!"

"I will never have an abortion, & I will never allow my daughter to have one. NO ONE that I care about will EVER have one!"

With that, she turned on her designer heel, & stalked out, her embarrassed daughter bringing up the rear.

What do you think about the story you just heard? Do you identify with Ms. PC? -- or maybe with her daughter?

I told you her story for a reason: Ms. PC couldn't be a better example of a VERY large chunk of America. Let me explain: Her daughter attends a pretty expensive Catholic High School & she's a senior. That means Ms. PC & her husband (if she's not a single mom) have been paying tuition for 4 years to a school they know teaches their daughter that abortion is wrong. If Ms. PC attends church, she probably tells her priest that she believes abortion is wrong --- so, emotionally, she's Pro-Life.

BUT ---- & it's a HUGE "but" ---- she STRONGLY believes that it's Every Woman's Private Right to Choose, so she's politically Pro-Choice.

And there you have it ---- the heart of America's Split-Personality Psychosis on Abortion: "Emotionally Pro-Life & Politically Pro-Choice".

------- Wow. Two diametrically opposed viewpoints in the same brain. Impossible, right? --- OK, now let's be honest--- unless you & your family are actually in the Pro-Life community, I'll bet that's exactly the way you'd describe yourself -- am I right?

And that's why every time the A-Word comes up, you just want it to GO AWAY. It gives you a giant headache just to think about it. Of course it does --- just look at the big split right down the center of your brain --- we're talking Migraine-type headache. Relax, I've got the cure. Read on.

In these pages, you've discovered a Great Truth:

ABORTION HURTS WOMEN !!

And if you're anything like Ms. PC, you're really ANGRY because you know that women have been LIED TO FOR DECADES ----- & WOMEN DESERVE BETTER !!

Here's what I think happened after Ms. PC & her daughter left the auditorium that day: I think she began telling everyone who would listen about this awful thing she'd just discovered called PAS. She told everyone, but most important, she really impressed it upon her Inner Circle -- all the people she loves. If Ms. PC or her daughter or any of her vast network of family & friends find themselves pregnant, there will be NO abortion ---- Adoption may happen, but it is certain that baby will live ---all because Ms. PC will not allow herself, her daughter, or anyone she loves to suffer the slow death of PAS.

Here's what I think is happening in Ms. PC's world today: At social gatherings, if the A-Word is brought up, I'm sure she still loudly proclaims herself to be Pro-Choice.

But then, if the person she's talking to is someone she respects, or cares about, she lowers her voice, & tells them the Truth -- what she knows about PAS -- & then she probably says something like the words I overheard at an upscale cocktail party: "Of course, it's your Private Right to Choose, but if I were you, I'd choose not to subject myself to PAS --- after all, it's only 9 months, & adoption is so easy these days".

How do you feel about smoking? You have a legal right to choose to smoke --- but knowing what you know about lung cancer, why on Earth WOULD you? If you smoke, I'll bet you're trying to quit. If your teenager wants to start smoking, I'll bet you move Heaven & Earth to make sure they don't.

------- How is this different??

How is "You've Come A Long Way, Baby" any more a LIE than "My body, My Choice" ------???

THE LAST STORY

In the beginning, I said you would hear 6 stories. You've just heard Story# 5 --- Ms. PC.

I can't tell you how the 6th story ends, because the 6th story is yours. I know a little bit about you:

If you're a male, you're the husband, father, son, grandson, nephew, brother, cousin, uncle, or friend of someone who's Post-Abortive -- or maybe you are post-Abortive yourself (PA fathers have their own kind of PAS) -- or you are both of these.

If you're a female, you're the wife, mother, daughter, granddaughter, niece, sister, cousin, aunt, or friend of someone who's Post-Abortive, or you are Post-Abortive yourself --- or you are both.

No matter which of these describes you, one thing is certain --- you are one of us. At the end of this book, you'll find lots of ways to access lots of information, help, & support for all of the millions of us.

Think back to the first story you read -- my story. Remember I said that, while the details of the story are mine, the main points & the broad strokes could belong to any of the 3300 women who stand outside that door every day. ---- and if that woman turned to face us, you would know her.

So who are you? ---- You are me --- or someone close to me. ---- & now you know the Truth.

I don't believe in "accidents" or "coincidences" --

There's a Reason why I wrote this book & there's a Reason why you read it.

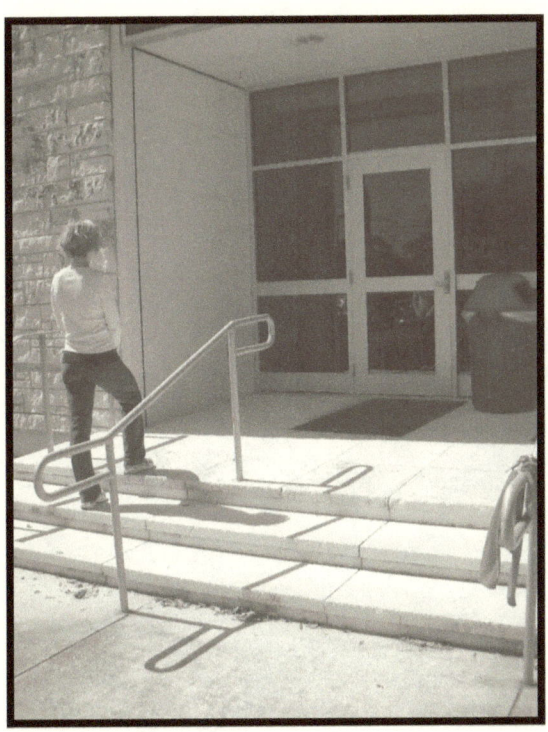

--- HERE'S THE INFORMATION I PROMISED ---

#1 --- Go to: national right to life. org/outreach

#2 --- Click on "American Victims of Abortion"

#3 --- Click on "Post Abortive Help"

Here's just some of what you'll find:

Association for Interdisciplinary research in Values & Social Change (Post-Abortion Syndrome, PAS research)

After Abortion (broad source of resources)

Project Rachel (links to Project Rachel & Rachel's Vineyard Retreats, etc.)

Bethesda The House of Mercy (excellent support resource)

Fatherhood Forever Foundation (general information & help For men)

Reclaiming Fatherhood (more services for men)

Breast Cancer Prevention Institute (excellent breast cancer information)

ProLifeInfo.org (general info & good list of complications)

Option Line (support & assistance for pregnant women)

Silent No More (opportunities to share public testimonies)

Her Choice (real audio clips of PAS testimonies from women & men)

Priests For Life (healing & help from many sources)

Ramah International (lots of PAS info & help)

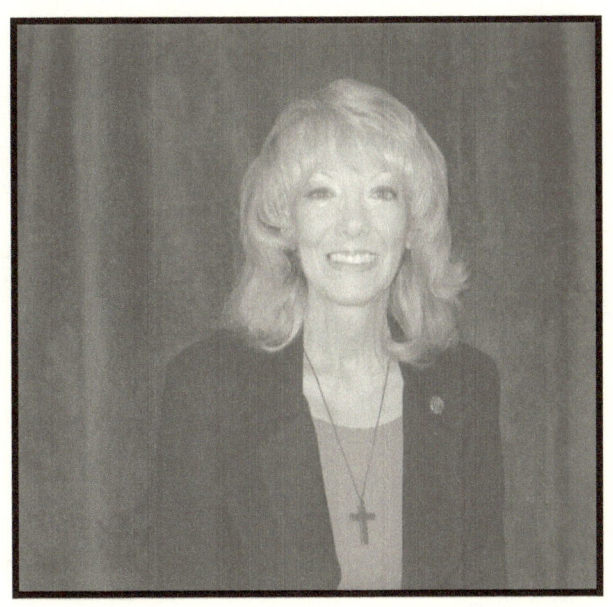

For the last 13 years, Vera faith Lord has traveled the country and the world, speaking and educating on the devastating effects of Post-Abortion Syndrome. She is a nationally published writer and a truly effective speaker. If you've ever been in the audience, you'll never forget what you heard and felt.

--- CONTACT ME ---

Go to cmgbooking.com

Go to authorhouse.com

Go to verafaithlord.com